I0492533

Self-Healing

Master Your Life:

Learn Powerful "Energy Healing" Techniques,

Holistic Healing, Mindfulness &

Affirmations

New, Updated and Improved – 3rd Edition

Chris I. King

Respective authors own all copyrights not held by the publisher.

Legal Notice:

Disclaimer Notice:

is not engaging in the rendering of legal, financial, medical or professional advice.

By reading this document, the reader agrees that under no circumstances are we responsible for any losses, direct or indirect, which are incurred as a result of the use of information contained within this document, including, but not limited to, —errors, omissions, or inaccuracies.

Table of Contents

Introduction

Thank you and congratulations for choosing to read my book, *"Self-Healing."*

This book contains some great and exciting information on how to heal yourself through powerful Energy Healing techniques, Holistic Healing Mechanisms, and Positive Affirmations.

The 21st century has brought about great technology, science, and medicine, but we are still prone to the primitive nature of various diseases and illness. Whether it is cancer that spreads throughout the body, small rashes that form, or even a runny nose, these ailments are very much a part of our lives. Diseases have evolved over time and so have our approaches and outlooks on healing them.

But are surgeries and pills the only way to beat the disease and sickness? Is there no way to escape the chemical cures that surround us? We must remember that before the evolution of science, there was a time when people used natural healing as a cure for their physical woes. In those days, they turned to the method of self-healing. Where your mind, body, and soul are all very much a part of the healing process.

If we are to believe the words of the great Greek physician Hippocrates, then "Natural forces within us are the true healers of disease." This book will attempt to uncover the meaning and validity behind that quote. I hope this book will guide you through a step-by-step process of self-healing.

This book will empower you with the ability and belief that you can heal yourself and give you a chance to become the captain of your own ship. We will explore the idea of psychological, social and spiritual stability as a cure for your sickness and hope this book will be the guiding light.

Thanks again for getting this book, I hope you enjoy it!

Before we begin, here is a small GIFT for you from my publisher as a thank you for buying this book.

The Ultimate Beginners Guide to Yoga.

What is Yoga?

Why is Yoga Beneficial?

What are the different kinds of Yoga?

What are the different types of Yoga Equipment and Accessories?

Get answers to all your above questions in this FABULOUS book. Reap amazing health benefits.

Please go to the below link and download for free

https://shininguniverseenergy.leadpages.co/beginners-guide-to-yoga/

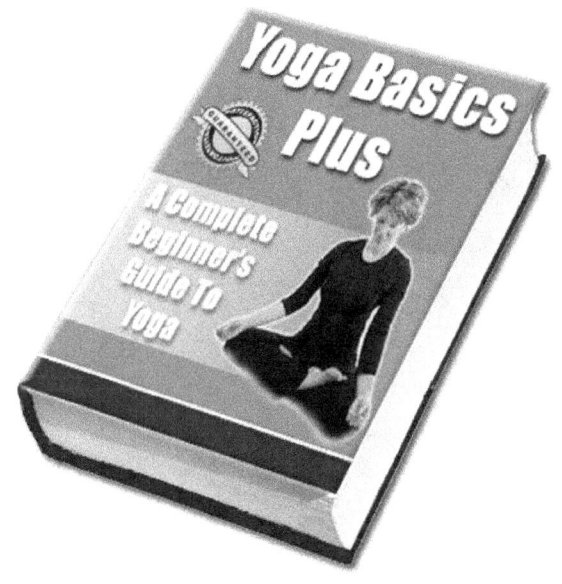

Hope you like your gift. And now let's begin our
topic on 'Self-Healing.'

Chapter 1: Belief In Self - Healing

Faith is having a belief or a trust in something. Take religion, for example, Hinduism, Buddhism, and Christianity, basically the world's greatest societal entities, exist because of the faith of people in different ideologies. Faith and belief are those qualities that drive one's motive (which in itself is a major asset to the process of self-healing). The purpose of this chapter will be to establish that foundational, unquestionable and unflinching faith in the power of self-heal so that you can do your best to achieve it.

So what does it take to establish such strong belief in self-healing? It takes conviction and some amount of truth.

Before we go into the logic behind this practice and why and how you must believe in the power of self-healing, let's first define the true nature of self-healing. The term in itself is quite self-explanatory, to begin with. It is the act of healing oneself. In life, we have to face countless hurdles in the form of a disease, illness, psychological disturbances, and trauma. People of all ages; from infants to elders, find themselves trying one way or the other to heal their physical or mental anguish.

Self-healing incorporates the idea of the mind, body, and soul into the process of recovery. Every pain is one that forms primarily in mind. If it weren't for our brains, then none of what is going on in our physical body would be recognized. So while our minds are the ones that form the pain and bear it, our souls have the ability to transform that pain and interpret it to a feeling. Disease brings along every kind of pain and suffering, and this is only possible because of our souls. Remember, as British Novelist C.S Lewis once stated, "You have a body and are a soul."

Our ability to feel things related to our body comes from the soul and mind. Self-healing calls attention to how the mind and body are two sides of the same coin. They are inseparable, and by treating them as two different variables that have an effect on each other, you are saying that your mental and emotional state impacts your health, and your health impacts your mental and emotional outlook. A tiny example of this would be the difference in treatment of the same illness between a patient who has depression and one who does not.

So, why would you even consider self-healing in the 21st century when you have the luxury of doctors and medicines? While the method may seem unconventional, it boils down to the most basic and simplest of life's hacks. Clinically speaking, it is the validity of the mind-body relation that should drive you towards this process. An example of this is a case where a patient diagnosed with MPD (multiple personality disorder) was allergic and bore symptoms of insulin-dependent diabetes while exhibiting one of their personalities and showed no such symptoms as the other personality. Another interesting story is that of another patient whose menstrual cycle changed every time her personality did. This shows that people experienced different reactions in the same body. This happens because the thoughts you have affect the type and amount of hormones released into your vascular system. Hormones, in turn, are chemical messengers that affect the way your organs act. Even scientifically, it is your mind controlling your body rather than the other way round.

You might have heard people say that the main difference between a good doctor and a bad one is their attitude. So what do people mean when they say that? It is said that a good doctor can heal your ailments even before he prescribes any medicine. This happens because the doctor is comforting and reassuring. He makes you believe that he will heal you. He affects your mind in such a way that you become calm and positive about the illness or ailment you are facing. If you can make yourself believe in positivity and self-healing, you can perform that same major psychological impact of the doctor, on yourself. Believe that you are capable of self-healing, believe that you deserve to be healed and believe that you will make it happen. You become responsible for the way you feel and the impact your body undergoes as a result of your optimistic thought process.

So when control can be exercised by the mind over the body, no matter how big or small your disease, there will always be some form of relief gained by self-healing.

Ask yourself why there are millions of people who are so passionate about yoga? Why mediation has existed for so long and why psychology is a science that people are studying? You may have heard of healers in South Asia who claim that they have always healed themselves through meditation and have never been to the clinic. Although this sounds impossible to us, many people have made it possible through their undying determination and belief.

I once met a man at a conference who said he had not been sick in over 20 years. I thought at first that this seemed like an incredible feat and maybe even a bit hard to believe, but I came to understand how he did it. He fully recognized the mind-body connection and used it to his advantage. He became attuned at detecting and anticipating when his body would be faced with a challenge and potentially under duress and was able to prepare for it. He didn't even wait until he saw signs or symptoms of a problem. He made a consistent practice of being mindful of his body. Through this practice, he was able to constantly fuel himself, heal himself, prepare himself and get needed rest. He saw his needs and he ensured they were met. He wasn't driven by external factors. In keeping his body and mind well, he was able to pursue his passions and carry on his life. At no point in decades had he been forced to give up a day or week to illness. It was hardly necessary to ask, but when I did prod a bit deeper for his methods and motivations, he was crystal clear. Not only did his practice of wellness mean he got to engage in each day of his life (i.e. not being taken out by illness), but he also got an incredible quality of life through his mindfulness along the way too. Quantity and quality both came through his personal practice. I was sold.

Anecdotes can speak to us sometimes. They help us see ourselves in another person's story. However, if science is your way to distinguish the truth you may even expand your knowledge and read through case studies of reported spontaneous remissions. From cancers, diabetes, high blood pressure, thyroid disease and much more. Every day, there are so-called "medical miracles" taking place. These will help give your outlook a paradigm shift. There are, in fact, patients recovering from diseases doctors has confirmed as incurable. These events may be miracles, but they also could be a product of self-belief and self-healing.

By now, I hope I have been able to establish in you some confidence over the self-healing method, or at least a curiosity. Confidence is important because with in addition to belief, there will need to be loyalty and faithfulness towards the method. This belief should be your reason not to give up, and continue consistently towards your goal. Another essential factor that comes with such valuable faith in the process is optimism. If you start out with the sense that things will fall in place, then they definitely will. Optimism is the quality associated with success and happiness over any other.

So with a strong belief in self-healing, a mindset that it works, and a positive attitude, you will be taking essential steps towards healing yourself.

Chapter 2: Mind Over Body

Buddha once said, "**Our life is the creation of our mind**." This is a thought to be taken seriously if self-healing is to be achieved. Changing our perspective and thoughts on our lives and our circumstances have great power over the way our physical bodies react.

In this chapter, we will focus on mindsets and affirmations to help you achieve a positive attitude. This is important because people often believe that a negative mental process can result in physical disease and turn, having a positive mental process can lead to physical healing. Take for example psychosomatic rashes; these are rashes that form simply due to mental factors such as stress and anxiety.

Our minds are full of thoughts. Your circumstances and environment have a big impact on the way you think. It is quite understandable why a person who is sick and not feeling well is in such a glum or somber mood. It is because of the illness in our minds and how quickly we associate it with morbid fears like suffering, death, and pain. The mind quickly resorts to the worst possible scenario and impacts our mood based on the fear of what could happen.

But what if I told you, that your disease is more than just a physical inconvenience? What if, your disease is an opportunity for you to learn and grow? When you are sick you become more aware of what is important and what is not. You can even take it as an opportunity to identify your true friends who will be there during times of need.

Physical or emotional illness can make you more aware of things you would otherwise take for granted. A friend's caring attitude or your pet's companionship. The sickness may present a chance to understand your weaknesses and the factors that make you vulnerable. The disease is simply a learning process and a part of life that teaches you the do's and don'ts for your body. Take this as an opportunity to learn and grow from it. Take it as your body is trying to communicate with your soul.

Remember that you are not defined by your disease, do not let it limit your opportunities and ambitions. You must simply realize that your disease is something created by your body and your body holds power to heal it as well. You are the creator, and you can become the destroyer too.

When you begin to identify with or as your disease or ailment, it holds on longer and stronger. Why could this be so? You would think no matter what, people do not want bad things in their lives. Most people don't think that pain or problems are desirable. At first glance, of course, they are not. However, there are benefits to pain. People may get attention for pain. They may get special treatment from others. They may be able to excuse themselves from doing things they don't want to do because of their disease. This is where the brain becomes miraculous. When you see a benefit to your pain, part of you desires it. Your brain can take a thought and make it a reality through your mind-body connection. Through your synaptic firing (your brain's activities), your brain can elicit hormonal and nerve changes that make the problems come about in your body. And since you get a benefit from them, you pay more attention and experience the problems even more. Studies have shown that when people retire, they almost immediately report a tremendous amount more health problems than when they were working. When studies went deeper, they found that people weren't having more problems, but rather having more downtime to notice their problems. So when you get some benefit from your pain, you can experience more pain because you are seeking that problem. You're shining the flashlight on it, and you will find it.

Incentives are also great motivators for healing. If you pay attention to the small things that make life worth living (your everyday routine, nature, friendships), then you will find reasons why you want to heal. It will ultimately make you appreciative of things and work harder to get back on your feet. Using moments of gratitude to get connected to what matters to you is useful. You bring to awareness the things that make you want to get up each day. By keeping these top of mind, you continue to build your motivation. You see more opportunities to try to heal yourself and stick with healing because you are so in touch with important things. You may realize how special people in your life are and then you get to thinking of the things you want to be able to do with them. Being well and living long probably ties in nicely with that, so the spike in motivation follows.

Changing your mental orientation to one that is optimistic, hopeful or future focused can help you along your journey to healing. Having a target in mind can help with the day to day healing. It especially benefits you if you can picture a future that you look forward to. You can use all of your senses for this. You can think of the feeling of being better. You may picture yourself in a specific spot, feeling good, the aromas around you, the sounds, even something you can taste. Being vivid with your visualization of your future helps make it seem that much more realistic. You start to create a mental model that you can live with. The thing about a vision for your future is that it does not just affect your future. Whatever vision you have for yourself is what you live for today. And if you haven't consciously created a vision, you're stuck with whatever your brain has created on autopilot. It is probably constructed of things from the past, maybe fears, maybe some things that excite you too and it is always with you. You may not even be able to see it as most people's autopilot mind is in their blind spot. However, it's there. So by taking the time to craft your vision for the future consciously, you are giving yourself a leg up. You are crafting what you begin living into today.

You can also begin planning for the future out of your visualizations. You can translate all of the good ideas, feelings, and hopes into actionable steps. You can start getting specific. When you get specific, you can begin to take action today toward achieving something. It may be small, but bit by bit over time you surely start moving toward that goal you set for yourself. When you are sick, you have plenty of time to think. Why not use that time to think of positive things vs. the physical sickness? You can use that time to understand your desires and make plans for your future. Think of the places you want to visit, or the new friends you want to make, the new foods you want to try, the adventures you want to take and the amazing things you want to accomplish after you are healed. Your dreams can act as a huge incentive for you to get better. Your plans will excite you and uplift you to the point that you find it unacceptable not to get better.

People say that laughter is the best medicine. Laughter has been proven to be a very effective medicine indeed. This adds to the evidence of the mind-body connection. You must also be open to laughter and the idea of letting it heal you. Let go of the inhibition that holds you back from laughter. Forget political correctness, morality, and even diplomacy for a while and give yourself a little laughter. Many say that laughter is the shortest distance between people. So even if you feel silly to laugh sometimes, chances are it only bring you closer to those around you. And it also allows you to be a space where laughter happens. You serve others through your laughter. You teach people laughter is okay and even encouraged around you, which further builds the amount of opportunities for laughter that you experience. Surround yourself with people who make you feel good. Don't be afraid to be silly. Keep an open mind and don't be afraid of being judged. Remember that you have one life to live and that it is best to live by your guidelines, not someone else's.

There are certain aspects of the body you must always remember. Your body knows how to heal itself. The self-healing process is natural in the body. Cells are constantly growing and dying, and the body has a way of maintaining and restoring itself. Think of all the bruises and cuts you've acquired and how over time they have vanished. Merely imagine the thousands of white blood cells fighting off bacteria within your body. Every cell, every tissue, every organ in your body is constantly working to revive you to full health. Listen to your body and your intuitions and trust the signals they send. And remember to honor those messages, because not even the doctors always understand your discomfort and pain as well as you do. Often our bodies send us subtle signals before larger ones. When we start to feel tired or we get a small pain, it is often a smoke signal to tell us to take care, slow down, rest and so on. When we practice mindfulness of our bodies to notice these things, we have access to care for ourselves early on and not let the problem escalate. When we stay too busy and distracted with the outside world so much so that we miss the signals, or we decide to power through them in order to serve some other goal, we often end up much worse.

Remember that the very structure of the universe will collapse without you here and now, and that is how important you are. Your presence affects the present state of the earth and the world. You affect people's lives, whether directly or indirectly. You may have saved a person from an accident simply by stopping to ask him for directions. That person may turn out to become the president later. The possibilities are infinite; you just never know! You play such an important role in the universe. You may not understand your significance yet, but you should keep believing that you serve a very unique purpose here on Earth.

Another aspect of divine alignment that is useful to understand is the brain component. We interact with the world through our attitudes, beliefs, and opinions. We create reality because we expect something and do actions that align with that thing being so. When we meet someone who is unstoppable in their pursuits, sometimes we think "that can't be done." For us, trying to find a solution to something huge might be a feat that we would not pursue because it doesn't seem likely that a solution can exist. But none the less, they keep at it. They see the world in such a way that the solution they are seeking is there, somewhere, waiting to be discovered or invented. And because they keep pursuing, they eventually find it. So their beliefs and their mental orientation did shape reality. Our beliefs that something can or cannot be done has everything to do with what is and what will be. When we have opinions about our bodies and what is possible, we take action in alignment with that. We seek more help if we think a better solution might be out there. It's not always a direct path, but we often do find a better solution.

I met a woman whose husband had about ten years previously had a stroke. The doctors told them that he should stick with rehabilitation for a year. The doctor warned that after a year, anything he had not recovered would not be improving moving forward. So the couple had worked through rehabilitation for a year, made some small gains and then accepted that nothing more could be done. They had resigned to the idea that the doctor was right and that was that. However, a few years later, the man met another stroke survivor who had stuck with rehabilitation for five years and continued to make gains to have mobility, dexterity and balance improvements. This was very encouraging. In fact, the new research shows that stroke survivors can even make new gains after years of not even trying to make improvements. Once they get back into some type of rehabilitation or growth program, so much is possible. Sure enough, the man started a plan to try new tasks each day and month by month was improving in all of the metrics that mattered to him – strength, balance, independence and language too. His new mental orientation that recovery was possible was entirely the foundation for this. So it's not just that you wish for something and the universe brings it to you. But no matter what you think is possible affects your everyday activities and decisions. Accumulatively, over time, these small things add up to your reality and your path. This plays out very tangibly in your health and healing.

It can also be helpful to think about a body-mind connection and not just a mind-body connection. They are, in effect, the same thing, but sometimes language can help us frame things in a more astute way. So in thinking of a body-mind connection, we begin to see how the state of our body can help our mind. This is a loop of body-state to mind-state and back to body-state. Take, for example, putting your body in a state of physical joy. This could relate back to laughter as I mentioned above. So create a circumstance where your body is laughing – either through humor, jokes, sharing with a friend or something of the like and then watch your mental state start to shift. Then use the new mental state to help you deal with any physical healing you need. So you've intersected the loop by consciously putting the body in a good situation which has come back around to help the body overall.

The practice of laughter yoga, created by Dr. Madan Kataria in India is based exactly on this. He realized that, as a general practitioner, he had many patients who relied on pills to deal with small everyday problems. He knew people needed some outlet to help themselves be well without relying on this practice. He started researching the health benefits of laughter for a medical journal article he was writing, and it donned on him. Laughter is good medicine. He began inviting people to a park in Mumbai to tell jokes and laugh. That worked for a long time but as the group ran out of jokes, so too did they run out of laughter. So he started a practice of laughter exercises with no jokes needed. He simply would give instructions to exercise, just like doing any exercise at the gym, and then people would follow. So he got people laughing for no reason except to laugh. The health benefits ended up being the same as "genuine laughter" – that is laughter that happens in response to something funny happening. This was revolutionary, and now laughter yoga happens in dozens of countries around the world. People put their bodies in a state of joy, their minds follow, and their bodies are stronger, healthier, more resilient as a result. Research shows that people have a higher personal immunity to cases of flu by engaging in laughter. So this body-mind connection can be critical to conceptualizing the importance of establishing a stellar physical and mental awareness and sense of control or ability to shape and change.

To further help in the self-healing process and facilitate a healthy mind and body, many people use affirmations. Affirmations are merely positive statements that we tell ourselves that are proven to have a positive impact on the subconscious mind. The most effective affirmations are those which are positive but also believable. When they are unrealistic, our brains grind a little bit trying to reconcile our uncertainties and current beliefs with the new ideas we are saying. When we put ourselves in a positive mindset to generate useful affirmations, we choose things that are optimistic and perhaps not yet entirely the case, but still within arm's reach enough that the affirmations motivate us and inspire us.

Here are a few examples of self-healing affirmations:

- I deserve to be healthy.

- My body is healing itself.

- I am ready to be healthy.

- I choose to be happy and healthy.

- I take care of my body because I love being healthy.

- I am a growing and changing person.

- I am capable of healing.

- I am in progress toward being my best self.

- I am healing each day and becoming stronger.

- My body is clearing itself of any problems.

- I am letting go of being ill and committed to feeling better.

- I am experiencing my body healing itself.

- I am experiencing health.

Because your body is so well attuned and each part carries out its daily tasks in rhythm and harmony. By telling your mind how you want your body to react can only enhance its functions and keep it working in a healing direction. It's this positive self-talk that keeps us on track with our micro decision-making too. So if we know we need to lose weight as part of our healing process, by affirming ourselves as healthy people through some of the above-mentioned affirmations, we might make better food and exercise decisions. When we reinforce to ourselves that we are healthy, we might not reach for a second plate of food or drive instead of walk. We will be more likely to act in alignment with that way we see ourselves – healthy.

Repeating these statements out loud every day has been a proven to heal the body and improve our overall mental attitude. Use the list above or make your own affirmations for whatever your situation is and the language that best resonates with you. Remember to make them realistic and well-fitting to you. Someone else's affirmations may work for them, but they do not necessarily work for you. Take your time to play around with language until you get the right fit. Getting into a daily habit of using affirmations will help you in your self-healing journey and move you further toward a positive mental state.

Chapter 3: Exercises For The Conscious Mind

So far, we have discussed the best perspectives that the mind must have in order to practice self-healing, however, those are only theoretic concerns. They are mere reminders and statements that are for reading and implementing our minds. If we are to approach self-heal more pragmatically, then the mind must be exercised too. Ways must be adopted to give your consciousness things like relaxation, freedom, and strength.

But how do you tap into such deep depths of your mind and exercise a smooth control over it so that you can, in turn, control your body? You can start by giving self-hypnosis a try. Here, in order to make the unconscious brain more susceptible to believing various ideas, you use open suggestions. As the mind may sometimes rebel against your direct instructions hypnosis will be a great way to take the other road to change. In hypnosis, once a person reaches a heightened state of focused concentration they are most likely to express a change regarding thinking, habits, and control.

To do so, you must first prepare yourself for hypnosis; whether that is through comfortable clothing, a quiet room, an isolated environment, or figuring out the goal of the hypnosis. Once you are completely relaxed, it will be time to enter hypnosis. Close your eyes and release yourself of feelings, fear, stress or anxiety. You may also recognize the tension in your body, take slow, deep breaths and lastly, enhance your hypnosis by testing yourself physically through exercises, visualizing different situations and using external guidance like music, sounds, and timers to lure you into a trance.

The most important thing, however, is to use self-hypnosis to better yourself. If there is a bad habit you'd like to kick out of your system or a new quality you would like to see in yourself, then hypnosis is your tool.

You might think of self-hypnosis as a type of consciousness raising exercise. Another word for it is meditation. So it's not just about convincing yourself or tricking yourself into something. It's also, more simply put, bringing awareness to yourself and your body. Meditation can be various things to different people. The theme is always awareness. And through elevated awareness comes the potential to do anything with our minds. We can break bad habits that affect our health. If you have a bad habit of snacking in front of the television, awareness can change this. Instead of just doing your routine of grabbing food before you sit down, by bringing awareness to it you also bring decision back to it. You reintroduce choice. You can ask yourself if consuming 4000 calories at night in front of the television is what you choose to do. Of course, old habits die hard, so it's possible that you still struggle with changes to the habits, but you get a whole new access to choosing to drink tea or have a better alternative snack instead. You can easily see how this awareness raising has a direct impact on health. So any meditation practice – whether simply noticing the breath or doing a mindful walking meditation can help you develop these awareness skills. Anytime you can pay attention, be in the present moment and add in choice, you are building your mindfulness muscle.

Another technique to heal your consciousness is externalization. This is an exercise of unconscious defense mechanism. It is to project your own internal characteristics onto the outside world.

Our body is sometimes so full of emotions, thoughts, and inner sentiments that it becomes too kaleidoscopic a view to sort out. We function in such a way that we are always searching for truths and needs. When we cannot do that, we have a feeling of total ambiguity that washes over us and anxiety takes over. As an ill person, you let your sickness and "what ifs" cloud so much of your decisions that you are confused and washed over. The solution to this is always externalization.

Externalization calls for activities like writing, talking or even pretending to be someone else. These are activities that are a great release for such energies. Say you have past experiences you want to free yourself from, or secrets about yourself that are too burdensome to keep. A way to free yourself from these loads is the old fashioned way of writing a letter or keeping a diary. However, do it without the fear of judgment. When you write, think that no one will ever be able to read what you have written. Write without constraints or fear of grammatical incorrectness. Write down whatever comes into your mind and thoughts, even if you feel like they won't make sense to others. Do what you may with it when you finish pouring out your thoughts and emotions, tear it away if it gives you solace, hide it away or never come back to it. But the point of it all is to come to peace with those thoughts and yourself.

If writing is too much of a task for you, then try talking to a chair! As crazy as it may sound you may talk to an empty chair and pretend as though someone, in particular, is in this chair. If the idea of sharing your problems with others is uncomfortable to you, just talk to yourself! Be your own best friend. Let your controversial thoughts interact with each other. You can even use different puppets and give each one a different voice and opinion and personality.

This will help you figure yourself out and figure out your stance on the problem.

Or perhaps give your anxiety an identity, detach it from yourself and give it its own name, features, and characteristics. Interact with it and figure out its problems. Then, help it figure out solutions and care for it so that by the end of it, you are taking care of anxiety as a person and in turn taking care of yourself.

While the two techniques mentioned above are solely under your control, there are also things you can try out with the help of others. One such practice is psychotherapy.

A psychiatrist, psychologist or a mental health provider may do psychotherapy. Here, different techniques are tried out in order to treat your mental health. You may be asked to freely associate, where you pour out all your feelings and thoughts, or you may even have to answer some questions. Such facilities are available in most towns, and most sessions are conducted hourly. Given the confidentiality of the session, you must interact with the person freely and truthfully so that you get the best treatment. If you like, you may even do this in a group or pair so that there is someone else there to relate to.

You might even want to try joining a support group recommended by your psychiatrist. Interacting with people undergoing the same problems that you are can help you emotionally. It will make you understand that you are not the only victim of your problem and that you do not have to go through it alone. You will be able to share your problems more openly too. Furthermore, you may receive advice from people who have undergone the same sorts of difficulties that you have. They will have been in your shoes at one point in their lives and will be able to empathize with you more powerfully than others. They can act as pillars of support for you and as examples that you too can succeed and get through the trouble like they have.

There is also the powerful technique of visually guided imagery. Various clinics have practitioners of this technique. Such people help evoke or generate mental images of various scenes that simulate or recreate the sensory perceptions. You may even have to use a recorder or visual aid or script to facilitate this healing. The imaginative or mental content experienced usually precipitate strong emotions or feelings. This could be a forest, the sea or any other place in the world you consider a safe haven full of comfort and relaxation.

This process usually requires a different institution; at home, you may try another type of visualized healing. This requires you to visualize in a quiet environment so the actual biological and physical healing of your body can begin. Say, you have lung cancer, before surgical procedures or medication take some time to visualize a clean, healthy lung, free of cancer and functioning smoothly. Spend minutes, if not hours, thinking about everything from the color to the linings -- everything. This is a very active way to stabilize nervousness that stresses the mind while on medication.

Coaching is an alternative to therapy as well and is sometimes a better fit for people at certain times in their lives. Life coaching, wellness coaching or other types can take a person-centered customized approach to help someone get something they want. Coaches often work with people to transform thought patterns that lead to undesirable life circumstances. They often work with people on goal setting and visioning for the future as well. They also can add in accountability for someone to stick with their new wellness plan. So coaching has elements that therapy may add, but it is more growth and action-oriented often. All coaches do things a bit differently, just like therapists, so ask around and see the right coach for you.

What I want for you to do is pick at least two of the techniques mentioned above and routinely practice them at least once a week. Remember that you must always conquer the mind first, and laid out for you above are ways to do that.

Chapter 4: Metaphysical Energies

Metaphysics is the study of the basis of all religions or ideologies in the world today. It works under the concept that bad energies or negative thoughts can cultivate illness and diseases into a person's physical body. Metaphysical healing is the belief that there is a definite connection between the body and the mind and that one cannot work well without the other being in a balanced state. Another great concept to understand about metaphysical healing is the fact that everything has energy- a pen, a bird, a plant, a tree, a door, a dog, a person- everything! Be it animate or inanimate, all of their energy derives from the same source, and as in the laws of physics, this energy can be transferable. Energy is everywhere, but it is up to you to filter and take in only the positive energies. This isn't too hard, though, thankfully!

Now, it is important to understand that the mind and a person's psychology work greatly to accelerate or slow down the process of healing. As I have mentioned above, reassuring doctors are also people who work under the idea of metaphysical healing. It is all psychological, but at the same time, it can evoke major changes. Metaphysical healing encourages your spirit to heal your body. Only you can make this healing happen.

A great way to practice metaphysical healing is to sit and point out what it is that worries you. This will help you heal because often, the type of disease you have relates to the worry that you have in your mind. Although this may sound ridiculous, studies have shown that people with money problems are more likely to experience lower back pain. Sometimes, feelings of anger, sadness, and guilt also work to incur pain in different regions of the body. Therefore, it is important first to get to the root of the problem. By eradicating the root, you can get rid of the disease as well.

Two main questions that metaphysics want you to ask yourself are: 1) Ultimately, what is there? And 2) What is it like? For you to heal yourself, it is important for you to know how you understand the concepts of nature and life. You will understand then that what you think and how you think will shape your life on a daily basis. In accordance with this, you can make alterations in your life to give rise to positive thoughts that can improve your overall health. However, you must also be accepting towards the views of others and also be able to see things through their eyes. This leads to more thoughtfulness and empathy within your soul.

Metaphysics has several laws that I will state in brief here:

The Law of Forgiveness - "We cannot be forgiven until we forgive others."

The Law of Attraction - "Thoughts are things and whatever you think about you attract into your life."

The Law of Substitution- "It is impossible to eliminate a thought from your mind unless you fill the space with something else."

The Law of Intention- "Whatever you intend to happen will happen."

The Law of Cause and Effect- "Every cause has an effect and every effect has a cause."

The Law of Freedom- "A person is responsible for all of his or her actions, thoughts, and energy patterns happening in both the seen and unseen worlds."

When you can understand and apply these principles, you get the most benefits from metaphysical healing. This technique does not require any experts or professionals. It is something you can do and apply in your daily life. In time, it will help you develop positive relations with others, clarify your mind, gain what you want and ultimately help you heal.

Take time to review the above list and then work with it a little. You might speak with someone else about your ideas about it, write about each in your journal, research them online or simply meditate on them. So go one by one and give time and space for each. Concoct ideas in your head. Think about how these may have each played out in some aspect of your life before. Think about how you can harness the power of each to your advantage with your health and healing. They each may be very powerful for you, or maybe one speaks to you at this time, and another will feel more important later. Don't get hung up, but be sure to take some time to massage each for its value in your healing process.

Chapter 5: Healing The Soul

Healing the soul is often a complex topic. Because what is it really? The soul isn't something that you can see. It is merely what you are within your body. Your soul is your true self, your identity, or your spirituality. Were it your body, you would have medicines and ointments to use to heal it should it become sick. But no medicine reaches the soul. Healing the soul is something only you can help yourself with. Now, you must understand that every soul has female and male energies. The female elements include nurturing, healing, calming, expression and emotion. The masculine energy encompasses logic, reason, action, firmness, survival, common sense and ease of acquiring material needs. In today's world, we find that we have given the latter much more importance than the former. We have begun to prioritize materialistic things more than the things that nurture our soul. Time and again, it is important for you to rejuvenate the soul by being in contact with your feminine energy.

So what can you do? Start out by understanding yourself. A great way is to undertake meditation. For at least thirty minutes at the beginning of every day, try to meditate. If that isn't possible for you, go to a quiet spot and think about life, think about you. Think about your desires and what your soul wants. For those thirty minutes, stop thinking how you are going to earn money or what you are going to do to make your next business plan work. Make it a time where you stop worrying, and just take a minute to be grateful. Think about the amazing gift you have been given- the gift of life, of nature, of sensations, of feelings, and of freedom. Embrace the unique soul that you are. Even among the seven billion people in the world, there is no one else exactly like you. You being alive makes a difference to the whole world. Think about how valuable you are; about how significant every soul is. Every alteration to a soul can create a domino effect. Each soul can affect another. It is really a beautiful phenomenon. Take the time to think about this beautiful process. How does it happen? Who made it happen? Why is the world like this? Everything has a purpose. What do you think the purpose of your soul in this world is? Take it all in little by little.

Go throughout the day and attempt to spread love, support and gratitude. The best way to do this is to help someone in need. Go to the orphanage and donate something to the children. If that is not possible for you to do, then learn some new activities and teach them to the children. Kids are excited about every new thing. Try to bring some innovation and purpose into the activities that you make them do. Teach them something that is bound to help them in the future. They are sure to be grateful for it in time.

You could also just show kindness through small acts. If you see someone having trouble crossing the road, help them cross. If you see someone grumbling and arguing with themselves, reach out to them and talk it all out. Help him clarify and find solutions to his problems. Compliment people who seem sad. Make everyone aware of their importance, of their significance. Help boost their self-esteem. Encourage them to do great things. You, yourself will begin to feel encouraged. If you have stray animals in your neighborhood, give them some biscuits if you can't adopt them. Go to the animal shelter and interact with the animals there. They will be radiating love and warmth towards you, which will work to help heal your soul.

Perhaps you could even visit the local church, temple, mosque or general place of worship. Regardless of which religion you follow, you must understand that every living being and soul has derived from the great source of energy which we have named God. Try to be in oneness with him. Understand that he is the origin of all life and of the things you see. See wealth as nothing more than just a worldly pleasure and understand that that is not the most important aspect of life.

You must also try to recognize that you are one of the small drops that constitutes the ocean of life and that all beings, all souls are interconnected. We affect each other in miraculous ways, but we affect ourselves in an even greater way. You can heal yourself by just being you. There is no one else like you. Learn to accept yourself. Let go of any past sins, regrets or mishaps. This is not a race. Take your time with this. Be warm and loving towards yourself. Do not judge yourself for being sick or wounded. Rather, love your vulnerability. After all, it merely proves that you are still human in this world that has become largely robotized. Embrace your emotions and the way you feel. It will help you understand your soul. What you like and what you don't. What is suitable for you and what is not. How you want to be, what you want to achieve, what aim you have in mind.

Wounding and healing is just a regulating process. Things like this are natural, and they take time. Believe in yourself. Try to find balance within yourself. Try to cultivate neutrality within yourself and learn to be happy. When you can do this, there is nothing that can disrupt your internal happiness and your internal peace. When you attain healing, the soul becomes an automatic process.

To accelerate your soul healing process, try to relax yourself completely. You can do this by taking hikes to new places, listening to the songs you like or by performing activities that you like. Once in a while, treat yourself to a relaxing massage or a spa day. Do everything you can to fit into your body and into this life. It will give you time to think about your life while your body has the chance to relax as well. It is definitely a win-win situation.

Another great way to understand and heal your soul is to recognize your passions and likes. In this day and age, your passions have been obscured by worldly obligations- be it duties towards your family, your work, your institution, your friends or even your house! Try not to think about your responsibilities, but just be in muse with your passions. Forget the lack of wealth or capacity. Imagine doing the thing that you love the most. Do not starve your soul of the passions that nurture it. Find out what your heart reaches out to and if you haven't found your muse yet, go and try out new things. How are you going to discover your passion for paragliding if you have just watched it on television and never actually tried it? How will you realize how talented you are at ballet if you never give yourself a chance? Disregard everything that anyone else might have criticized about your passions. Only you can judge what will benefit your soul. Make a bucket list for the things you want to try. Then go out and try them out! If that isn't possible, the best thing to do is to imagine and visualize you doing those things? Do you feel glad? Scared? Excited? Exhilarated? Annoyed?

If you have been meaning to take a new step in life and turn over a new leaf, it is bound to have you worried. It keeps you anxious and wondering about the future. This deprives your soul of balance and integrity. So you know, the best thing to do in this situation is just to take that big step. If you have planned it for a long time and it seems right, there is no reason to back away. Believe that destiny has marvelous things in store for you. Think positive and work positively. Unlike magnetic poles, in this case, positive attracts positive. When you cultivate positive energy within you, you will be attracting positive things, good things and unimaginably wonderful things. Now, many people would translate this as "sheer luck." But that is not so. "Luck" is simply something that follows people who believe in themselves, in the greatness of the world and has the belief that destiny will make their dreams work out little by little.

Now, I have told you all this, but you must understand that the single best thing you can do to achieve all I have mentioned above is to prioritize your spirituality over everything else. Learn to take time out just for yourself. Turn off your phone if you have to. No materialistic possessions or even jewels are more valuable than your soul. Take time to accessorize yourself internally rather than spending hours trying to live up to society's standards of beauty. Nothing is more important to you than yourself. Although that sounds selfish, taking care of yourself should be everyone's priority, and you are not wrong merely for understanding that.

Chapter 6: Modifications to Life

A great deal of self-heal is also about making modifications to what you are already doing, but not doing right. Your lifestyle is an essential aspect of healing yourself and self-heal requires you to make various changes to even the simplest of routine things in life. Remember that the only reason you feel unwell is because you might not have habits that benefit your body. Take sleep, for example, the single most taken-for-granted activity whose magnificent impact is yet to dawn upon many. When you sleep, several important hormones release into your bloodstream. Your body is finally getting a chance to use its energy for healing and not functioning. If you do not let it rejuvenate itself properly, then everything from your mood to stamina will be affected the next day. By sticking to a sleep routine of at least 8 hours, you are doing yourself a huge favor and building subconscious positivity for the next day. Furthermore, sleep also helps to boost your immunity, which in turn primarily keeps you from becoming sick. Before sleeping, you must also unwind a little through active thinking or meditating or exercising so that you leave all of your stress aside and indulge in good quality sleep. Needless to say, you must also focus on your achievements of the day and positive things to give your mind the rest that it needs. Think of all the good things that have happened to you that day count your blessings every day!

Nourishing your body regarding nutrition is also imperative. You are what you eat, and if you do not eat right in this age of carbonated drinks and excess sugars, then you are putting both your body and your future at great risk. By this I also do not mean following a strict diet plan that will bring down your weight or give you a flat tummy in weeks; these are unrealistic and have an expiry date. Your lifestyle, on the other hand, is forever and therefore your goals with nutrition should also be realistic. Meaning, you can and should never really cut out all the fat from your diet, instead, learn to distinguish between good fat and bad fat like the fat found in fish and avocados vs. fries and cheese. Incorporate more green to your diet and increase your fiber intake. Cut down on empty carbs and processed food, and substitute them with whole grains and lean meats. Also, remember to drink up to eight glasses of water daily. Look through World Health Organization's recommended dietary goals if you must, they will provide you substantial guidance. Learn to plan a well-balanced diet that works for you, rather than merely skipping meals.

Undertaking some relaxing, but, effective activities for your health will also be beneficial to you. Yoga is a great way to bring about flexibility and freshness within you. However, if you think that yoga isn't for you, you can opt for meditation. The true purpose of meditation is to rejuvenate every single cell that constitutes your body. It will help cleanse your mind and keep it free from worldly worries and problems, albeit for a short period. It will refresh your body and mind. Additionally, it works to cultivate positive thoughts and incorporate positive energies into your body. It also fuels relaxation and healing.

If you struggle to get yourself into an exercise regimen, ask yourself what is missing that has it not happen. This can be very revealing about what motivates you. It may be fun that is missing. So you know you should work out, and you got your gym membership, but you hate going. Over a short time, you don't even set foot in the gym. On the other hand, however, you love swimming, and you love hanging out with your friends. Heading down to the community pool is way more enjoyable. It may not be as perfect for your weight loss or strength building as weight training, but you sure look forward to it and get yourself down to the pool a few times per week. You added fun, and your behavior around it changed. You're going! Sometimes community is missing. When you add in a buddy who wants to walk with you or a friend that wants a little friendly competition to stay active, you've got yourself a recipe for success. So look for what is missing and discover what really gets you going. Once you pinpoint it, ask yourself how you could meet that need (i.e. add in that desirable element) so that the exercise happens. And if you first think that there is no way that you will enjoy exercise, then challenge yourself to come up with ten possible ways that you could meet that need with exercise. Find 10 solutions. Be really generous with your brainstorming and then also give yourself a chance to experiment. Try a new class. Check out dancing. Try being outside. Borrow a friend's equipment or ask them to show you their favorite sport. Explore, expose yourself to different things and keep an open mind for finding the joy in something that maybe always looked like a drag to you.

When it comes to daily activities, I would also like for you to incorporate the idea of rest between your activities too. Take a break of fifteen minutes or so and just relax from your hectic schedule, this will open doors not only to fresh spirit and energy but also brings about the flow of ideas and creativity. Something close down this line is also the act of reducing stress. It is important that your body focuses on healing and recovering rather than stressful work. So for the moment being, I also advise you not to undertake any such work, and instead perhaps take a long overdue vacation.

Your attitude will also play a major role in the process of healing. Maintain a calm composure even during difficult times, because stress only works to throw you off balance even more. No matter how pressurizing situations get, maintain a sweet, polite tone. If you find yourself boiling over, definitely take a break or moment to yourself. Move your body. Get that moment of respite with fresh air. Change it up so you can let your mind find peace or at least form coherent thoughts instead of being a victim of your emotions. This keeps you away from frequent arguments and helps build new relationships. This also leads to lesser conflicts and a clearer, more relaxed mind.

If you find you get stuck on rails where you get stuck escalating your anger or frustration after it rears its ugly head, then you can practice these techniques. Sometimes all we need is a moment to derail our thinking to keep ourselves from getting really angry or frustrated. Because your mental space is so important to your healing, it is worth figuring out the best methods for you that will allow you to be effective in your self-care in the short and long term. You and your body deserve it.

Follow the breath – the great thing about any meditation or practice that involves the breath is that we always have it with us. We need no other special equipment. We can employ breathing techniques at our jobs, in a meeting, in traffic and anywhere else. Breathing is always acceptable. Plus, it only takes a few minutes. Simply shift your attention from whatever the situation at hand is to your breath. When you ground yourself in your body and ground yourself in the present moment, often we gain perspective on the circumstance. Our minds don't sweep us away and race. We get back to a calmer state and become more capable of dealing with whatever triggered our mood or emotion in the first place.

Count to 10 – This is a simple yet effective technique for pausing any emotional situation that is escalating. You simply count to 10 in your head. Once you break the natural trajectory of automatic reaction, you give yourself a chance to take a new course. It removes the moment of acting from a place of seeing red, being scared or being reactive. You can do this with children too. Count aloud and let them experience the process of slowing down for a moment and being able to think before acting.

Draw your experience – We often are called to action by our emotions in the form of verbal or physical activation. We find ourselves wanting to say something, scream or act out physically. Drawing is a great way to express ourselves. It is especially useful if we feel strong emotions but cannot articulate them in words yet. Drawing takes out a mental filter, so we can express something without needed to find words. Then once we draw, the process often reveals to us the critical aspects of the experience and why it is so emotionally provoking.

Physicality – Being able to release our energy in a physical way -- can be so calming. First, it's raw and invigorating and expressive and then it is over. If we channel our emotions into a burst of physical activity, we get to pour out our cup of emotions if you will. A sprint jog is good for this. So are jumping jacks, dance, pushups and the like. Maybe just 10 seconds – 1 minute will do the full trick.

Find someone to embrace – As bizarre or maybe animalistic as it seems, hugging is helpful. We all started life inside a squishy, comfortable, warm and safe place – a womb. There is something still relaxing about any moments that recreate such an experience. If you establish some people in your regular environments that are comfortable with a hug, this can be an excellent tool for you. If course, it can also be a tool for connection, not feeling alone and giving a little boost to another person too. But primarily in this context, it can be seen as a way to calm ourselves down and regroup emotionally.

Take a moment of self-care – Over time, and as you build your personal awareness, you can identify the things that you can do, say or be that allow you to regenerate energy and find peace of mind. For some, it is being outside. For others, it is connecting with someone you feel safe and happy with. For others still, it may be doing something creative. A lot of people like healing activities.

Create comforts – Create comforts are the habit side of self-care. Sometimes they are not the healthiest, but they still allow us to dissipate a tough situation. Ideally, they are in the realm of healthy. Create comforts are those little things we go to when we want to feel in control, relaxed or comforted in some way. Food, cuddling in a blanket etc. may all fall into this category. These are our defaults that we find ourselves naturally drawn to. Taking a moment to fall into a habit can help shift us out of a negative trajectory that was headed some place much worse.

Shift gears – When we find ourselves in a situation where we are determined to tackle the problem head on, and we start getting really rigid and stubborn about it, we probably need to switch gears. This is not natural to do, but absolutely effective. This can mean changing our environment like physically going to a new place and doing something new. It can also mean shifting our thought patterns at the time. For example, you can switch from a moment of frustration to a moment of learning. That's a real mental shift. You can't stick with your pattern of negativity, frustration and so on if you are actively trying to learn something new. There are many applications for your phone and computer that can be perfect to shake up your mental space. Language learning apps that involve games can be very accessible in a time like this because they take just a few minutes, they are easy to jump into, and they often have some level of challenge or fun. The consuming nature of learning helps break our mental trajectory. Doing a physical learning moment can also be helpful. Back in the 1980s, it would be common for people to have a physical puzzle on their desk. It might be a metal object with moving parts where you had to separate two parts. It wouldn't be easy to figure out, but that was the idea. Take a moment from hard work or frustration and just learn and play physically for a moment.

Get it out – Our minds are constantly processing the outside world. Our minds are generating opinions, ideas and beliefs about everything happening around us. Whether or not our thoughts are rational or even based in reality is beside the point. Our minds will consistently generate in order to try to make sense of the world. The trouble comes when we grab onto thoughts and relate to them as reality. That is why it can be good to process those thoughts before taking any action on them. Writing them down is wholly effective for processing. You can write yourself a journal (on paper or digitally) where you say everything that runs through your mind at that moment of frustration. Write what you think about what happened, the behaviors you witness, the injustices you have seen, how you think things should go and even your possible courses of action. Sometimes journaling can help make clear what the next steps are. Other times, writing things down simply allows the individual to release emotions without having social recourse. And once these things are written out, then their emotional hold over a person simply disappears. It's amazing how that works. Another way of writing something out is to write a letter to another person. So this is not a carefully crafted letter that rationally states the situation and solutions so that you can get a certain result or figure something out with another person. It is actually a letter that just dumps all of your ideas, emotions and says everything completely unfiltered and ultimately frank. This is a letter you will not be sending. The process of writing it to another person can be satisfying, though. And by releasing all that you have to say to that person in the frustrating moment through a letter, you somehow help yourself put water under the bridge and get on better with that person.

Take your pick from the above menu and try them out. It is helpful to choose a default. Since we're not always at our best in moments of frustration, it is best when we know our coping strategies and can employ them without too much thought or processing. As we heal ourselves, we are bound to run up against frustrating moments. Even when we're not in the process of conscious healing, we know that negative emotions left to run will do harm to our health. So having healthy methods to deal with emotions is positive for our health and healing overall.

Chapter 7: Physical Pursuits of the Body

Although this chapter sounds nothing short of superficial, you'll be surprised to know that it actually isn't at all. In fact, it once again centers on the argument of the mind-body connection. Many say that your body hears everything that the mind says; however, the body itself can work on many ways to heal itself. Such manual exercises are those that shall benefit you both mentally and physically.

First, to start off, meditate for at least twenty minutes daily to reach a state of "thoughtless awareness." You must cease all thought process through focused awareness, especially on breathing as every breath signifies your vital energy. Another thing to keep in mind is to be still and release all your mental stress. Meditation is perhaps the simplest form of exercise for the body that can reduce stress and anxiety and enhance creativity. It can also improve various things like memory, blood pressure and reduce pain and risks. Now meditation can be hard to get into if you put too much pressure on yourself to completely clear your mind. Meditation is a practice, and there is so much to be gained out of the practice and not just achieving a clear mind. In fact, people who meditate for years do not have a completely clear mind. What they do have, however, is a trained ability to acknowledge when they have started thinking and then decide just to let the thought go. That is, in fact, what meditation is. It's the movement through focusing on the breath, setting an intention to clear the mind, noticing when thoughts arise, peacefully dismissing the thoughts for the moment and returning to the breath. You may find thoughts popping up constantly. You've just planned your next week during your meditation and then when you realize it, you think "I've done something wrong." Absolutely not. You are fine. Simply notice what happened. Don't make yourself wrong. Simply return to your breath. All is well. Meditation is a transferrable skill because things constantly pop up in our lives and being able to see our challenge with them and then peacefully dismiss our unwanted thoughts about it or our unwanted behaviors is a meditation practice. The two parallel each other nicely. So it is not helpful to try to have only a clear mind because our lives are never clear, making the practice

78

non-transferrable. Be generous with yourself. Don't focus on being perfect or trying to get better. Meditation is not about getting somewhere. It is about witnesses the here and now in whatever that is. It is about practicing un-attachment to what comes up in your thinking. You are not your thoughts.

If you are to take meditation a step further, then yoga is another practice that has been universally popular and well accessible. Go to your nearest fitness center or hire a personal instructor for the best results. This includes you doing both bodily exercises like stretching, working on posture and building strength as well as mental practices like controlled breathing, and relaxation. Through yoga, you are expanding the flexibility of the mind and that of the body and restoring balance on both. Some yoga poses to kick off with would be the triangle you stand with your feet apart and keep both legs straight as your torso hinges at your hips toward the left leg as far as possible. The Surya Namaste is also a well renowned wholesome package that you can repeatedly use for building strength. The great thing about yoga is that it also has a wide range of growth, meaning that there is a beginner's level, a level for amateurs and an advanced level, so there is plenty of room for development, and the practice could serve as a recreational delight too. There are hundreds of websites available that provide instructions, poses and even videos about how to do yoga. Doing just a few postures can be a very healing practice. Balance postures are super for grounding yourself in the present and developing body awareness. When you are doing something physically challenging, it always helps your mind from racing too. You are called by your body to be fully present in the moment. You cannot multitask because your brain is needed to care for your physicality. You are needed to be aware of everything around you to be able to balance and stay upright. Tree pose where you stand on one leg and place the other foot on the inside of your thigh (or calf) is straightforward but calls on you to find balance.

There also various other healing exercises that have different cultural roots, like Qigong, which is an ancient Chinese holistic system of healing. It typically involves moving meditation, wherein you perform Qigong sitting, lying down, standing or moving. Obviously, the difference in these types leads to different oxygen intake and additional body movements too. It brings a new dimension to meditation, as repetition is barely a focus here. Instead, the three corrections of body posture, deep rhythmic breathing, and calm mind regulation. Qigong is timeless, and healing may take place in a split second. When you perform the exercise is also a matter of personal preference. By coordinating slow flowing movements of different forms, Qigong has been said to improve a wide range of medical conditions including hypertension, pain, and even cancer.

A martial art turned healing exercise that is similar to Qigong is Tai Chi. It is also known as "meditation in motion" or "medication in motion." Here, you practice a series of low impact, weight bearing and aerobic movements that improve your physical and mental health. Again, due to its methodical feature tai chi must be learned through a trained instructor of some sort. It is a great way to reduce pain and stiffness and even enhance sleep. It also helps to maintain balance and posture. These slow, considered movement shift us away from the rushed and busy attitude that we are often plagued with. We learn to slow down, be present and practice mental awareness.

Acupuncture can also be used to treat emotional problems. This once again sheds light on the fact that the body and the mind are interconnected. This traditional Chinese healing technique believes in an energy form called the "Qi" which is said to travel throughout the body. When the body and mind undergo emotional pain or other emotional distress, the passage of Qi becomes obstructed within the body. By using needles to puncture the skin, acupuncture attempts to unblock the passage of Qi to relieve the person from their emotional pain. Although many may not believe in this treatment procedure, Qi is in fact just a metaphor for the metabolic processes of the body, and the process of acupuncture shows promising results. A study published in the Journal of Acupuncture and Meridian

Studies gave students a 20-minute acupuncture session. These students then showed to have better memory and lower levels of stress than other students who hadn't undergone such sessions. Therefore, making use of acupuncture is also something that you can do to heal your soul. It normally does not hurt and is a unique and relaxing procedure that is gaining popularity day by day.

Reiki is another astounding healing therapy. It is based on the principle that the therapist can transfer energy into the suffering person through touch. This then creates a domino effect and accelerates the natural healing processes of the sufferer himself. Now, you may be wondering how to find a Reiki master for yourself because this type of therapy is quite rare in several parts of the world. The best way to approach this would be to search for advertisements in papers, or even easier-search online! Now comes the more difficult part. How do you choose which master is the most suitable one for you? You can do this is by evaluating his qualifications to make sure he is certified. Also, check his experience. Try to choose someone who has successfully treated many patients before you. Check his knowledge and make sure he knows every small detail of Reiki and his check his branch of Reiki. Reiki has many categories, so you must make sure your master has studied the type that you require. Also, when searching, try to find out what he will teach to you for the fees he charges so that you can opt for the best deal. However, keeping in mind all of the above, make sure you follow your intuition because only your inner self can recognize the master who can successfully heal you. Ultimately, choose the master you feel most comfortable with!

Almost any kind of healthcare can be generative to you and your healing. Touching as part of your care can be particularly useful in creating the notion that the body is healing. This reinforces further decisions to heal the body and choose generative activities, food, and habits. Chiropractic and massage are two excellent ones. They both involve touch and are healing-oriented in their very nature. You can feel the end of healing through these processes because pain and blocks in your body are addressed. Your movement may become less restricted. You may feel more energized and lit up about life. Your body may feel taken care of. Being touched can also help you understand your body better. Through interaction with a health care provider, you can feel new sensations which reveal different things about your body and what it is dealing with. It can also be encouraging over time to have many treatments and physically experience what it is like to physically improve. You may feel it when someone's hands are on you. It doesn't feel the same as it did last time. That pain has subsided. I feel much more relaxed. Noticing these changes can be reinforcing for your health journey. Invite these kinds of experiences into your life. If possible, find time each week to do something in the realm of physical healing. This is good in the moment, but it also helps you build momentum toward having a good health trajectory in progress.

If seeing a practitioner is not something you can or choose to access, there are many alternatives. A 10-minute session in a massage chair at the gym or mall can help with your healing and sense of relaxation. Sitting near a jet in a hot tub can also provide a similar experience. Even palpating yourself or your pain spots with your own hands can provide some benefits.

To relieve your body from all that negative energy and exert that energy outwards, stick to one of these exercises consistently. Make it a goal to master it; weight loss might be a perk, but the overall sense of calm and relaxation is the ultimate deal.

Chapter 8: Environmental Adjustments

A major reason for illness is often an unsuitable environment. Sickness might be your body's way of telling you that you are not in the right environment. In this context, the term 'environment' does not merely encompass things such as cleanliness of air or the availability of clean water. What is also important is your social environment and your surroundings.

It is important to stay in a healthy physical environment. Try to keep away from polluted, crowded areas because these are often home to several pathogens. To heal yourself, you must first calm yourself down. To do this, I recommend that you find yourself a quiet spot that you can walk to every morning or at least during your free time. Breathe in long, fresh breaths and watch the sunrise. Morning time is when you can fully observe the beauty of Mother Nature. Close your eyes and immerse yourself in the lovely sounds of chirping birds, the smell of fresh air and the feeling of being alive. Cleanse your mind of any grudges or past regrets that you might have. Every morning begins a new day and every new day can become a beginning to a new, healthier life. Recognize how lucky you are to be part of this beautiful world and think about how lucky this world is to have you. Brisk walks can also help to keep you healthy and away from future ailments. Try to keep this up every day.

Appreciate of beauty should not be understated. There is something innately generative about being around that which we find to be beautiful. For some that is nature and for others it is art, but find what yours is and don't forget it. The arts are a wide field, and there is so much beauty to be discovered. I recently visited a small town in a farming belt that seemed at first glance like it was devoid of the arts. Then someone invited me to check out a play happening at a small theater on the outskirts of town. I didn't have high expectations, but I was curious, so I went. I was blown away by this small ground of amateur actors who did quite a moving play. I find that to be beautiful and I felt very energized as well as peaceful after the play was over. You can find art galleries all over. Even art shops can provide a moment of respite where beauty abounds. Take these moments to heart. Make sure they happen. When we drain our cup, we must refill it. When we are facing health challenges or feeling depleted in some way, witnessing beauty can help us refill our cup. Nature is full of beauty. Just think of taking a few minutes to watch birds playing together, building a nest or feeding their young. These things may happen around us all of the time. In turning our attention to such beauty, we get to be engaged in the act of curiosity and appreciation. These are helpful states for our mental and physical wellbeing.

I read a blog of someone who recently returned from Iceland. They had been having pretty consistent migraines in their day to day life and were struggling even to consider taking a vacation. They had always been captivated by the photos of waterfalls and fjords, and so they just took the risk and made it happen, not knowing if their trip would be plagued by migraines. They felt a little uneasy on the plane ride to Iceland but as soon as the plane was descending and the incredible landscape began to appear, they felt their heart warm. They described the beauty that they found at every turn. They hardly wanted to sleep because it was so nourishing to be around such raw beauty. They became very much aware of what it meant to witness and engulf themselves in what they found to be beautiful. Not once during their trip did they get headaches. It simply did not happen. They wanted too much to be able to be outside. They took care of themselves so they did not have to miss out. And each new beautiful landscape only helped them feel more and more well.

Once in a while, try to take a vacation and go to places that you have never been to before. It doesn't always have to be to another country or another continent, maybe just going a few bus rides away will do the trick. This will inculcate fresh and out-of-the-box ideologies into your mind and will keep you from just thinking about your sickness. Go to places that make you happy and that soothe you. They will further aid in the process of rapid healing. Novelty and discovery can be captivating experiences. When we are captivated, we turn ourselves over to an experience and sometimes find ourselves refreshed and renewed on the other side of it. Travelling provides this is mass amounts. Not only do we see new things like architecture, different people, natural landscapes, and new art forms. But we also hear new languages, music and the sounds of a new urban cadence. We taste new things like spices and beverages. We may feel things like a breeze on our skin, the heat of the sun or a kiss on the cheek from a new person (depending on the cultural tradition). Lastly, we can stimulate our sense of smell by baking food, sniffing flowers or even smelling unpleasant things like waste (by accident of course!). None the less, we are still captivated by these novel experiences. We often find new insights for ourselves when we fully embrace something new and get curious about it.

The curiosity and interest that comes from being in novel places, when embraced, can be harnessed into awe. Research in the field of positive psychology has found that a human experience of awe can be critical for personal satisfaction, healing, and happiness. Fully immersing ourselves in an experience so much so that we are amazed and impressed is the same as experiencing awe. You can see how traveling is a magnificent way for accessing awe. When standing on the edge of a canyon even deeper than the Grand Canyon in Peru's Colca region, visitors gaze up at the mighty condor as it passes. This experience of witnesses a huge bird in an inspiring natural environment is very much the perfect place to generate a sense of awe. When we travel, we often make an unconscious decision to look at the new environment with beginner's eyes. Think about when you first saw something. You looked deeply at it perhaps. You had a natural emotional reaction and over time that is not as automatic. You have gotten used to something. It is as novel or naturally awe-inspiring anymore. We look at things with more attention when they are new. We notice more detail. We can, however, bring these same beginner eyes to our everyday lives. If we make the conscious decision to get interested in an engaging way with what is around us in our regular environments, we might find awe there as well. This is generated within us. And while being in incredible and novel places helps us access awe more easily, we can become amazed at things we have even seen before. We might take a moment to allow for awe with people in our lives. Or we might realize that we walk by a park every day as we walk to work. Well, there could be immense beauty right there in our own back yards. When we bring our beginner eyes and curiosity, we get a whole new experience. Awe helps us with healing because not only are we more enlivened by any physically progress or healing that we make, but we are more creative and curious about the world. That maps right onto our personal healing journey. We seek more solutions, get more curious, and we feel more hopeful.

Sometimes, being around the wrong crowd may also affect the way you heal. Partying might be fun once in a while, but it isn't always healthy to be doing that every day. Also, try to stay away from drinking and smoking because these are bound to hamper your health. Do not indulge in activities you do not like simply due to peer pressure. Rather, try to be around encouraging people who genuinely want you to heal as fast as you can. Such people will take care of you and keep you away from health hazards, as well as bad habits. These health allies cannot be understated. They become the best partners in getting on the right track and sticking with healing, even if they road is long or windy. If you have people in your life who are open to join you in healthy habits, that's super. However, if you spend time with people who already do those habits, then they're much more likely to be an effective ally. If they already go for walks or go to the gym and make good food choices, you can learn from and piggyback on their good personal trends. Spending time with them can only help you inculcate new, positive behaviors.

You should also try to surround yourself with people who are also trying to heal themselves and are not quitters. Find a few such friends and gather for coffee every once in a while. Talk about what you have accomplished and share your experiences with one another. Take advice from each other about methods that have worked for you. Cooperate and work together.

94

After all, as Helen Keller once said, "Alone we can do so little. Together we can do so much."

Support groups, when done well – even informally – help people to be boosted in their health, healing and recovery. People get to gain from each other's experiences and see what they may want to try themselves too. So it's not just hopeful that someone else was able to achieve something, but also people can share specifics. When you understand the specifics of something, it makes it that much more accessible to feel able to try a new solution. Speaking to someone who is in your situation and gained something is a great access point to new action.

The importance of the environmental health comes into play when we observe people who have healed simply by going to cleaner, more peaceful surroundings. Places with clean water, low amount of vehicles and more greenery are ideal for good health. This is because clean water means fewer microbes, and cleaner air means more oxygen for the body. More oxygen results in a greater supply to the tissues, and consequently, to a more active lifestyle. So try and find a clean, peaceful and soothing place to stay. However, I understand that this isn't always possible, so just try the best you can. If you cannot find a silent spot, try to plug in some earphones and listen to some classical music (or any music that helps you relax).

Clutter can also be harmful to our health. Having a cluttered environment can be both mentally and physically damaging. Regarding our mind space, clutter can bring about the sense that we need to do something, take care of something or simply bog us down in feeling overwhelmed. Physically, clutter can be harmful because we may inadvertently have poor air circulation, mold or constraints on our ability to move freely. This is on a spectrum for all of us. Sometimes we may vary in how much clutter we create and can handle. Marie Kondo, the Japanese clutter coach who wrote the book "The Life -Changing Art of Tidying Up" articulates the philosophy of clean living by encouraging people to have only the things in their lives that spark joy. She says that often people get overwhelmed at the thought of dealing with their things. Her rule is simple. Pick something up and if it sparks joy then keep it (and find the right place for it) and if it doesn't spark joy let it go. You can let it go to someone for whom it does spark joy. This takes the calculation out of the decision making and makes it so straightforward. Joy? Yes, or no. Done. By clearing our spaces, we leave room for ourselves to have peace of mind. This is so important when being on a healing path.

The environment that surrounds you plays a very important part in your health. It is essential to stay away from things you dislike, such as a boring job, an annoying acquaintance or unwanted habits. Again, it may seem selfish to you, but it is essential for soul healing.

Chapter 9: Simple Steps to Self-Care

Self-care is not something you achieve, and then you can just sit back. Self-care is a daily, weekly, monthly and yearly practice that helps you care for yourself over time and give yourself what you need to live a high quality of life as well as a probably higher quantity of life too. This chapter is about providing additional tools so that you can take care of yourself in a way that provides you the best possible life. Especially when we have some health issues, we need to be kind and generous with ourselves. Self-care is the foundation for personal growth and improvement in healthy people and those with health conditions alike. Some of the following were referenced or relate to other concepts and activities that have been shared thus far in the book. However, I want to be thorough and provide this in one place so you can come and grab a tool when you need it easily. When you are oriented to your health like you are the source of your solutions, you may find self-care activities become an essential part of your day. You seek them out. You prioritize them. You see the value, and you protect your time for yourself. You realize and embrace the notion that taking care of yourself makes all of the difference.

Life wheel – With health challenges comes a call to action to transform our lives in some way. We may be missing something in our life or have too much of another. By doing a bit of a scan of our life, one aspect at a time, we start to uncover and identify what needs our attention or adjustment. Picture a life wheel or you can picture a circle divided into pie slivers, and start thinking of the most important aspects of life. So people (relationships), romance, financial, career, learning, physical health and so one can go into your mental model. Now take each one and reflect on that aspect of your life. If you were to shade in that aspect of the wheel or pie, would you shade it all in to signify that you have a full aspect, meeting all of your needs and expectations? Would you fill it in half way to signify that you have many things going well in that area, but it is still not fully fulfilled? Begin with that visual and then build or unpack from there. Why did you choose that number to describe that aspect of life? What is working already? It's important to acknowledge what is already in place or functional in your life. What do you like about what you already have or have achieved in that aspect of life?

Then look at the space that is incomplete. There is nothing wrong, first of all. You are simply having a frank reflection of what desires and goals you have for yourself and what there is to be or do that will get you a fuller, balanced life (or life wheel in this example). So what is missing? What do you want in that area but do not yet have? What have been the hardships? Then gently explore the question of what can be done? Is there anything to be done or are you peaceful with where you are? What elements would you add or remove to that area of your life to have you be more satisfied with it? This is not a place for excuses. You do not need to defend anything or even be disappointed in where you are at currently. Just look for new opportunities for yourself.

In exploring this kind of generous way, you may find yourself getting excited or lit up about something new. You can inject that into your life which will not only bring you new results but bring you a new mental orientation right now. So by creating a new possibility, you shift immediately. Do this with each important aspect of your life. You may decide that a couple of things are priorities for now and other things will come later. Again, this is all in the vein of kindness to yourself. As you create new things that get your excited, your orientation to your health shifts. You are finding new things that may require your health to improve to pursue them, so you put more at stake that motivates you to take care of your health. When you have something worth healing, you can generate much more momentum toward healing.

Body scan meditation – I talked about meditation in previous chapters. It is an excellent tool for curbing negative mental patterns and finding peace of mind in any life circumstance. I talked about following your breath, letting thoughts go and keeping your mental energies on the present moment through a focus on the breath. Now I want to build on that and give you another tool for meditation. It's called the body scan because that is the main gist of it. You begin, like the other meditations, by finding a comfortable sitting position and begin to turn your focus to your body through watching your breath. Now you move on to do a scan throughout your body. You are not trying to accomplish anything, but simply do a systematic review of your body. Start with closing your eyes and move from the top of your head down to your toes in slow succession, experiencing and bringing awareness to each part of you. Almost put yourself outside of yourself to you can look at that part of the body, then feel that part of the body. You may notice different sensations like pain, heat, the feel of your clothes touching you or simply nothing. Often, we get so much into our intellect and heads that we lose a bit of the ability to notice what is happening in our bodies unless it is a mighty pain or extreme pleasure that calls us to attention. The practice of body scan allows us to return to a better awareness of and understanding of our bodies.

As you scan through, there is no need to adjust, move or fix anything that you notice. Just notice it. When you complete your meditation (after 5 minutes or as much as you'd like), you can explore more any of the sensations you experienced. Maybe you feel called to stretch a certain area, put on a sweater because you noticed feeling a bit chilly or even getting moving because you noticed energy inside of you. This practice helps with your healing because the more aware you are about your body and what is happening in it, the more you access you have to catch problems because they become big problems. Also, you become better aware at figuring out what helps and hinders you. For example, many people live in a lot of discomforts. They don't realize that some foods they eat cause unnecessary pain, bloating and gas. They just go about their day, eat what they eat and don't realize they could significantly improve the quality of their lives with a diet that better suits their bodies. And dietary issues can often exacerbate other health issues too. Through increased awareness practices, they become better able to catch these small things that they've just been stuck with for years, so much so, that they fly under the radar. They're just accustomed to not feeling well, so they are just resigned to it.

Moments of positive self-talk – I talked about affirmations earlier and even provided some examples of ones you might want to try or adapt in your path toward healing and full health.

Energy balance – If you want to be rejuvenated and capable of healing yourself, you need to look at where your energy goes in your life. What things build you up and invigorate you? What things fill your cup? Then on the flip side, what are the things that use your energy? Now this isn't an equation to figure what things to eliminate from your life. You may choose to do things that are draining because you want to help someone in some way. Or maybe that thing is challenging now because it is new or novel and you're not yet good at it. Eventually, over time, that same activity may become one that brings new energy to you. It is valuable to check in with this exercise from time to time so you can reassess. So you simply need a page and draw three columns.

On the left, you can simply write the list of activities you do in the run of a day. Or just choose yesterday for example. Write down routine activities that get your day started like, the visits you do with others, the different tasks involved in your work, your hobbies, your volunteer activities and so on. Then in the middle column write whether it is uplifting or depleting. Does it build you up or take energy? Again, we are not naming things to say that depleting bad and should be avoided. We're just in the process of being aware. Once you've done this, you can take any notes or jot down ideas in the right column. Like if you notice that the social things you do take energy and are depleting, you could note that. Or if you become aware that you haven't done much self-care, just jot that down.

Now review it and think about opportunities to improve your day. You may choose to complete the depleted things when you have the most energy in the morning. You may switch between depleting and uplifting activities so that you can constantly build back up your resistance and never fall below a comfortable and energetic state. You may also notice that you're only doing depleting activities for example. This may point to opportunities to add new generative things to your life or even more extreme things like change your living situation, job or health routine. You can decide to take one new action as a result of this exercise. You might call a friend who is uplifting and set up a time to meet them for tea. You could go sign up for the gym. You could decide to get more sleep. This exercise can help you determine new insights and actions that will help you along the glorious path to caring for your health and healing.

Creating you own self-care menu – We all enjoy a nice menu at a restaurant. Here we are already out to eat which is great because the hard work is done by someone else and we'll probably enjoy ourselves. Now we have the pleasure of perusing the menu to select that thing we want from a lot of great options. This self-care menu is much the same. We are going to generate a menu of things that are all good for you, feel good and boost you up in some way. When you are feeling a little depleted and too routine, you can select from this menu and treat yourself well. This is all part of building and maintaining great health. My friends do this great thing with their kids. They sat down and generated a whole bunch of ideas for rainy day activities. The kids hated not being able to go outside and play, so they made a game out of generating fun activities that they can do inside. They wrote each on a slip of paper, folded them up, put them in a jar and now when it rains, the kids are excited to pull an idea out of the jar. You could choose to add this element of surprise or simply make a list.

The self-care menu begins by considering what activities – large and small – build you up. Adult coloring books have recently become popular. Maybe that's an activity that is good for you. It can take a short or long period depending on what you have at your disposal. Maybe taking a bath or getting a massage is on your list. It could be as small as picking up your favorite treat on the way home from work. Think through the last time you felt calm, taken care of or joyful. Those of the memories that will help you uncover the things that are great to add to your self-care menu. The criteria for including things is really anything that makes you experience wellness in the moment, improved health, improved stress-orientation or calm. The things could be creative like art, self-expression, singing, dancing and the like. They could be physical like yoga, running, walking, swimming, biking, weight training. They could be playful like watching a comedy or looking at cute photos. They could be exploratory like learning about something that you've been wanting to understand better or experimenting with a new skill, among others like visiting a new place or trying a new activity. Self-care can be just about bringing immediate joy or pleasure like playing with a dog, engaging in kissing or a sexual experience or eating a decadent food. For many self-care means calm. So activities in the realm of calm or relaxing could include resting, watching a movie, reading a book, meditating, doing a spiritual practice, meandering through a park or so forth.

Hopefully, the above suggestions help you with generating ideas or jogging your memory about things that are self-care for you. Again, you get to define them. For some people, being in a social situation is uplifting, and for others, it is terribly draining and not resembling self-care at all. You decide. You don't have to "should" on yourself to only define self-care as going to the gym and drinking fruit smoothies. You can decide that artistic activities might be your source of joy and self-care. Generate your menu and decide whether you want to choose from your menu each day or have it in your back pocket for those times when you want to build yourself up. A routine of self-care helps build personal resilience and the ability to deal effectively with illness too so consider a regular cycle.

Play with feeling and touch – your sense of touch is amazing to explore when taking care of ourselves and putting ourselves in the present moment. Do a tour of your home just for a few minutes and look at the different things that you can experience in a tactile way. You may go to your closet and feel the different fabrics or linens. Notice what feels different about each – the thickness, the sensation and so on. Run water over your hands and feel the different temperatures. Notice changes to your heart rate to the temperature of the rest of your body too. Keep moving about and simply touch different things. It could be fun to make food that involved kneading or mixing by hand. This kind of exercise is short but can be great to ground yourself in your body and remind yourself how easy it can be to access a moment of pleasure with the things in your natural environment.

Be a tourist in your own city – I talked earlier about beginner eyes and what it means to see things with a fresh perspective, bringing a sense of wonder, interest, and even awe. It brings rejuvenation and helps us feel great and satisfied. Being a tourist in your city can be very convenient and bring you a sense of appreciation for your environment too. Check out your local museums. See the things that happen like concerts, festivals and outdoor activities. Visit the parks and look for the paths, statues and flowers that you normally just pass by. See them with beginner's eyes. Be a tourist. Bring your camera and set out to take photos of beautiful things. By donning that lens, you often see things you wouldn't normally. And the bonus is, the next time you leave your house, you get that warm feeling that you are surrounded by beauty because you have elevated the awareness of the beauty that surrounds you.

Edging to peace – Often we look at our lives, and if we see something that is out of place or not what we want, we think we need extreme change. And the prospect of extreme change can invoke fear and paralyze us from even getting started. This exercise helps orient us to make small shifts. It takes away the barrier to getting started by just thinking regarding edging toward something, not leaping. So start by considering the anchor points in your life that bring about the most stress or unhappiness. Now look at each one by one and generate a selection of "new futures" or possibilities for that thing. So if you think about being overweight and the moments where you feel stress because of that, generate ideas for how you would like it to be. Now instead of major transformation like going on a crash diet, consider one new micro habit that is in alignment with that goal. It could be something that involved a slight shift in what you are already doing. In the book The Compound Effect, author Darren Hardy offered the example that when someone switched from simply putting mustard on his sandwich compared to mayonnaise, he lost a fair amount of weight over just a year. It was such a micro change but he was able to maintain it because it was so accessible and doable. So this edging toward a goal can be a reliable way to move down your desired path. Go through each aspect of your life that involves unwanted stress and look for ways to edge toward your desires in that realm, making just small actions toward a better future. Having the new possibility in mind like being relieved or successful in those different realms of your life can help you conjure up these little actions.

Hopefully, these above tools will be of great use to you in your personal care work (and play). It is worth it to take care of yourself. You have a life to live and give. When you generate energy and take care of you, you can have so much more space to enjoy your life and to make a contribution to others too. If you're always just getting by, that's no way to live. Sometimes we need to do that for short periods of time because we want to accomplish something or we feel drawn or obligated to something outside of ourselves. But we cannot sustain this for too long without paying a toll. And remember, I am not just advocating for living without pain and suffering. This is not just a mission of living without any disease. It's about full health. It's about not just good, but great. Health is about adding what makes us most alive and minimizing that which diminishes wellbeing or finding a new way to approach things that do not compromise our health. Here's to your health.

Chapter 10: Embracing Self-Healing

Now that you have learned the several aspects of self-heal, it is essential that you wholeheartedly embrace it. Don't be afraid to admit that you are practicing self-healing, because there is no reason for shame. Instead, take pride in the fact that you understood that your soul was wounded and are taking steps to mend it. You don't merely have to stick to the techniques that I have recommended. You should also try to formulate newer techniques if you feel like they work better for you. The key objective of self-heal is to understand yourself, your significance and your purpose. Self-healing is not something everyone is open to, but don't let that discourage you. Different things work for different people. Even your own identical, genetically similar twin can have different likes and dislikes so if people that you hardly know try to criticize you, disregard them. There is only one person who knows what is best for you and what will work for you. That is yourself and no one else.

So what are you waiting for? Go try out self-healing for yourself. Be your own physician. This doesn't mean eliminating getting the help you need and consulting people with expertise. However, it does mean that when you take the self-centered viewpoint or the responsible viewpoint that puts you at the center of your health, you become astonishingly more powerful at making a positive difference in your health. Take life events into your own hands. Become independent. Let your inner self-make decisions for you according to the way you want. Let things flow naturally and believe that every new day will bring you closer to becoming a healthy person physically, emotionally, mentally, vocationally, spiritually, socially and overall holistically.

If self-heal seems to work for you, teach it to others. It will be beneficial to people of any age group. It will help children develop into more confident, esteemed adults if they start understanding themselves spiritually from a young age. But this doesn't mean that self-heal doesn't work for others. It is never too late to begin self-healing, and it is just as effective - provided that you put in the amount of effort and determination that is needed. While helping and supporting others in this way, you are once again working to heal your soul. Supporting others in this away also keeps you in touch with the healing process. It will maintain your firm belief in self-healing which is another powerful aspect. Always understand the power of self-heal and remember what Robert Ingersoll very rightfully said once, "We rise by lifting others."

Chapter 11: Using Dreams to Heal Your Body

When you think about self-healing, there are probably several things that automatically pop up in your mind. Yoga, meditation and daily affirmations are most likely a few such things that your mind conjures up when the topic of self-healing is raised. One of the very last things that you would probably ever think of when it comes to self-healing is dreams. After all, what possible role can dreams play when it comes to healing your body? The fact of the matter is that the art of using dreams for self-healing purposes is something that goes back into ancient antiquity, having connections to various cultures over various times. While this art may seem lost in this modern era of medicine, the truth is that dreams are still used to heal both body and mind by countless people around the world. Anyone who can regularly remember their dreams will be able to easily use those dreams to help their body to heal itself from any ailment they might be suffering from.

One of the earliest and most primitive forms of dream healing can be found in shamanistic cultures. Ancient societies that had a shaman, or proverbial 'medicine man,' were renowned for using dreams in a great many ways. In these cultures, dreams were seen as a window into the spirit world. It was possible for an individual to visit with the gods in the dream state, something that was considered impossible while physically awake. Dreams could also take a person to distant lands, or even alternate universes, since the dream state was free of the physical laws that bind our waking lives. Another valuable application that dreams had in shamanistic societies was to help heal a person of sickness or disease. When conventional medicine, which usually consisted of herbs and animal parts, failed to do the trick, dreams were seen as the next step toward healing a person of their affliction.

The primary way that shamans used dreams to heal a person was to identify the cause of the sickness. We need to understand that ancient cultures had a significant knowledge of common illnesses and the natural remedies that would cure them. Therefore, whenever traditional medicines didn't work. the shaman knew that the sickness was something more than just a regular run of the mill issue. Since books weren't really an option, let alone Google, then the only way to find the solution was to tap into the Universal Consciousness, which was accessed through the dream state. In this scenario, the shaman himself would seek the dream that would either tell him the cause of the sickness or the source of the cure. Once the shaman had the dream they needed, then they could get to work making the medicine that would cure their patient.

Another way that dreams were used was in a more spiritual context. Ancient cultures often saw unusual ailments as an affliction of the gods, or as a demonic possession. By going into the dream state, a shaman could confront the god or demon responsible for the affliction and seek to end the sickness by appeasing the god or by exorcising the demon. Again, once the shaman was awake, they would have the knowledge from their dreams regarding what course to take in order to heal the sick person in their care. While this approach may seem like nothing more than a gimmick to us in our modern mindset, we should remember that a shaman only kept his position as long as he was effective. Therefore, these dream methods had to produce results, especially in order to have survived over the millennia to this very day. After all, shamanistic cultures continue to exist and thrive in different parts of the world today, along with the traditions of dream healing that every one of them possesses.

It is pretty easy to imagine primitive cultures using dreams to heal sicknesses and to 'cast out demons.' After all, what is a primitive culture without a half crazed medicine man or woman who is otherwise shunned by society? What may prove a little more surprising is to discover that some of our most scientifically and philosophically advanced cultures also used dreams as a source of healing for both body and mind. The most notable of these cultures is none other than Ancient Greece. One of the primary differences between the use of dreams in Greece, as opposed to shamanistic cultures, is that there is an actual collection of historical data accompanying the Greek experience. Everything from murals to inscriptions and even textual references can be found to describe the process of dream healing in Ancient Greece. Furthermore, these historical records go on to describe the *successes* of dream healing, listing the many ailments that were cured. These cures weren't the standard "I had a headache and now it's gone." type scenarios either. Rather they included such things as paralysis, comas, bad joints, sterility, and a whole host of ailments which had very real symptoms that could not be hidden. Thus, when the accounts say that a particular person was cured, you can bet that it happened. This is further demonstrated by the offerings that were made by the healed people to the gods, most specifically, the god Asclepius, who was the god of medicine. These offerings consisted of walking sticks, braces and any other medical aid that the sick person would be unable to do without unless their ailment was actually cured.

The use of dreams to cure ailments in Ancient Greece was not the sort of thing that took place down dark alleys in a hidden back room either. Instead, actual temples were dedicated to the process. These temples were called Asclepeion, after the god Asclepius, and they could be considered one of the very first forms of hospital to arise in western civilization. While not uncommon, Asclepeions were not always located in each and every city in Ancient Greece. Why they were located where they were is the subject of much debate, but what is agreed upon is that many people had to make a considerable journey to visit one. Unlike the process in shamanistic cultures where the shaman underwent the dream experience, in this case the patient had the healing dream. This dream could come in the form of a visit by the god Asclepius himself, wherein he would perform a miracle on the body of the dreamer, much like the miracles recorded in the New Testament. Other times the dreams would simply 'act out' the sickness and its healing, much the way dream symbolism often represents inner conflicts or struggles that dream therapists base their treatments on today. The important thing here is that the dreamer would wake up cured, as though the dream process had provided everything that the body needed in order to defeat the ailment.

By themselves, the examples of dream healing in shamanistic cultures and in Ancient Greek society may not seem like anything worth getting excited about. However, modern day research has shed light on dreams in a way that is still baffling many scientists. One of the most important discoveries is the symbolic nature of dreams. Researchers, including the notable Carl Jung, have revealed that dreams contain their own language, a universal language of symbolism. What is most fascinating is how dream symbolism seems to be universally shared, regardless of culture or religious belief. It is as though the language of dreams is spoken by anyone and everyone who experiences the dream state. This is significant because it points to a shared knowledge that dream symbolism is used to express. The idea that dreams contain a higher or deeper knowledge is critical for understanding how dreams can actually heal a person.

Just because the ancient traditions regarding healing dreams seem lost and left behind doesn't mean that the techniques won't work today. On the contrary, the universal aspect of dreams transcends time as well as space. Just as dream symbolism is virtually identical in every culture in modern times, so too is it identical over the span of thousands of years. This means that even though dream temples are hard to come by these days, healing dreams are not. The trick is to develop the ability to access and to use your dreams effectively. Fortunately, there are many traditions available today to help a person to connect with and make better use of their dreams. Such techniques as dream incubation and lucid dreaming are well researched and made available to anyone through such mediums as books, videos and even YouTube. If fact, the information available on dreams today may have made the ancients rather envious. If this information had been available in ancient times it might have been enough to put shamans and Asclepeion priests out of business!

The first thing to realize is that there are two distinct types of healing dreams. The first is the knowledge dream. Having a knowledge dream will help you to determine one of two things. First, it will tell you what is actually wrong with your body. You might find that you have symptoms that are either hard to describe or that doctors can't diagnose. Few things are more frustrating than a healthy CT scan when you know that there is something very wrong with your body. This is where the knowledge dream comes into play. Rather than relying on medical science to discover what is wrong with your body. you can use your dreams to let your body tell you what is going on. This may sound a bit over the top at first, but the truth of the matter is that there is a very strong connection between mind and body within dreams. And this connection can extend to actual communication through the symbolic language of dreams. After all, how else would you expect your body to speak to you except through symbolism? Thus, to have a knowledge dream is to have a dream where your body sends you imagery that reflects the nature of the ailment.

Many examples of this exist in case studies from around the world. One such example involves a person who was suffering from a mild fever and overall body aches. While these symptoms sounded like flu symptoms they didn't respond to flu remedies. After a week of no improvement, the patient had a dream in which he grabbed a red sponge like creature with tentacles and tore it off of his body. He threw it on the ground and shouted "Stop eating me!" The next day the person woke up feeling free of the sickness that had plagued him for over two weeks. Upon further analysis of the dream, the dreamer was able to realize that he had been suffering from an infection, and that the night he dreamed of defeating the red creatures was the night his body ridded itself of the infection it had been fighting all along.

This dream can be considered a healing dream as well as a knowledge dream since it involves the healing process as well. However, as it used symbolism to represent the nature of the infection that was plaguing the person it is an excellent example of a knowledge dream. The body knows what is going on, even when we aren't quite sure ourselves. In the case of this individual, his body knew it was fighting an infection, and it indicated as much on the very night that it was able to vanquish the infection once and for all. If this person had not woken up feeling better, they could have used the dream to determine the right course of treatment to help them to recover from their symptoms. In such a scenario the individual could have gone to the doctor and asked to be tested for an infection. Such a test would have turned up positive and the appropriate medicine would have been prescribed.

The other type of dream is the healing dream itself. The nature of this dream is that it causes the body to actually heal itself, requiring no additional treatments once the person wakes up. This was the type of dream experienced in the Asclepeion in Ancient Greece. Again, the dream example of the person with the infection is as much a healing dream as it is a knowledge dream. Therefore, just as the person dreamt that they overcame their sickness in the dream, so too would you expect to do so in a healing dream. Many case studies include such imagery as slaying monsters, dragons and the like.

129

Other imagery includes waking up from a deep sleep or some other image of growing in strength. Often when this type of dream occurs the result is that the body becomes strong enough to overcome the sickness in a short time after the dream. In any event, the important thing about healing dreams is that they act as a directive, meaning that the body either vanquishes the sickness or it begins down a path of recovery that is immediately measurable.

Knowing how these dreams work is only half of the equation. The other half is in knowing how to induce these dreams for yourself. Fortunately, inducing dreams is actually far easier than many people realize. This is especially true for anyone who already has a rich dream life. The main thing you have to do is to really focus on the dream that you want to have. You don't need to create the exact dream in your mind per se, rather you simply have to tell yourself over and over again that you want a dream about your particular ailment. This process may take several days to achieve, so it is critical that you remain focused and patient during that time. Many people expect immediate results from dreams, as though the dream process was similar to going through drive thru. What you need to realize is that the dream process is a deep form of communication, and this usually requires your mind to be free of all other preoccupations in order for it to unfold. Therefore, it is absolutely vital that you create a sort of mantra for yourself to repeat during the day, such as "I want to dream about my sickness." Needless to say, you need to choose the words that work best for you. However, once you form this mantra you need to fixate on it day and night until it produces the dream you need.

Once you have the dream, you then need to determine what kind of dream it was, one of knowledge or one of actual healing. If your dream is about seeing a doctor and having a specific conversation, or where a particular word comes to your mind, you have had a knowledge dream. It is vital that you record the knowledge immediately, lest it be lost like any other dream. Additionally, follow through with that knowledge as soon as possible. Go to the doctor and mention the word you dreamt of, or recreate your end of the conversation in the dream. It may be best, however, if you keep the source of your information secret, as telling the doctor you get your medical advice through dreams may have unwanted consequences... Sometimes the knowledge may come in the form of the medication you need or a change in diet. Many times a dream will involve specific types of food that will actually aid the body in recovering from its sickness. The important thing is to take the information seriously and to act on it right away.

In the case of a healing dream you probably won't need to do anything once you wake up. These dreams are usually ones that occur when the body has overcome the sickness or when the body starts down the path of self-healing. You can ask to have this type of dream when trying to induce your healing dream, and focus solely on self-healing rather than acquiring the knowledge of what it is that is making you sick. In order for this to work it is imperative that you firmly believe in the body's ability to heal itself. Any doubt in this area can significantly affect your ability to have a healing dream, meaning that it can take longer to induce.

Chapter 12: Understanding the True Essence of Sickness

When we think about sickness, we typically think about diseases, viruses and other nasty things that attack us from the outside. While this is a very real part of being sick it is only one aspect of sickness itself. One way to think about sickness is to liken the body to your car. To imagine that sickness is only about viruses and diseases is the same thing as imagining that the only way something bad would happen to your car is if you got into an accident. Sure, accidents will mess up your car and require a significant amount of work and expense to get fixed, but the fact of the matter is that most car repairs have nothing at all to do with accidents. The vast majority of car repairs are the result of components wearing out or failing for any number of reasons. Most of the time, these components are either well past their prime or they suffer from neglect, meaning that they dry out and break down sooner than they should. This is equally true in the case of sickness. Most of the time, sickness is less about exposure to a harmful virus or disease as it is about our body breaking down from age or neglect. Once we understand this, then our way of viewing sickness will change forever.

Most parts in a car require some form of lubrication in order for them to work properly. Oil is needed to ensure that the engine runs smoothly and that it doesn't seize up as a result of the tremendous friction and heat that it creates. Additionally, brake fluid is needed to ensure that the breaks work well, and transmission fluid is needed in order to keep the transmission from seizing and sticking. More often than not the first thing a mechanic will ask a person bringing their car in for repair is when was the last time they changed a particular fluid. The answer often reveals the nature of the car's problem. What any mechanic will tell you is that proper maintenance of your car will prevent the vast majority of wear and tear on the parts that make your car run. This will ensure that those parts last for years, meaning that you get the best performance from your car without any headaches or hassles. Additionally, taking proper care of your car will also affect things like fuel efficiency. The more run down a car, the worse the fewer miles it will get per gallon of gas. Alternatively, when a car is well taken care of then it will get the most miles per gallon of gas possible for that car's design. In the end, proper maintenance of your car will prevent many of the troubles that plague most car owners.

So, the real question is just how does that relate to sickness and the body? While the analogy of a car to the body can serve to demonstrate certain similarities there is one stark difference that makes all the difference in the world. That difference is that the parts that make the body work are made of living matter. All of the parts of a car are manufactured in a factory. They are made of metal, rubber and all sorts of inorganic material. As a result, the only thing a car part will know is decay and wear. Alternatively, the parts of a body are *grown*, not manufactured. This is a huge thing to consider, as it will make your understanding of sickness, and more importantly healing, vastly different to what it was before. The bottom line is that every part of your body grew to where it is today. We often think that once a part forms that it is done forming and growing and it simply starts to go through the same wear and tear as any part on a car. This is completely wrong. The fact is that the cells on every part of our body regenerate at a rate of every seven to ten years. This means that every cell in our body is no older than ten years old! Since our body rejuvenates at this rate naturally, why is it that we don't heal ourselves all of the time? The answer to that question is that we actually do. To demonstrate this fact, all you need to do is consider how your skin heals itself from every cut, scratch and scrape you ever encounter. The chances are that you take this process for granted. After all you have seen it happen countless times over the course of your lifetime. What you don't realize is that the same process occurs internally as well, the only difference being that you are usually unaware of it when it happens. This makes sense as you can't see your spleen the same way you can see your elbow!

If the body heals itself on such a regular basis, then how is it that the body can suffer from sickness and disease? The answer to this goes back to the analogy of the car. While the body is designed to renew itself, and even stave off sickness and disease, the fact is that it has to be properly taken care of. Unfortunately, most people don't realize just how delicate the human body actually is. While it can endure a great deal of use and abuse the fact is that the human body is a biochemical organism that requires a delicate balance of chemicals, hormones and energy. When these elements become unbalanced, the body's overall performance begins to suffer dramatically. Just as not changing the oil will cause your car's engine to seize up, so too, when your body's chemicals are out of whack you will be susceptible to all sorts of problems. Herein lies one of the most well kept secrets of sickness. The single most common cause of all sicknesses and diseases out there today is what is commonly known as stress.

In order to understand the nature of stress on the body you have to first understand the function of the brain. Many people think of the brain as being the seat of intellect, even of the soul in many cases. While this may be true, it is not important at this point. Rather, the chemical nature of the brain is what is critical for our understanding of how stress affects our physical wellbeing. The fact is that the brain is the electro-chemical command center of the body. Whenever you feel pain you are actually being told by your brain to feel that pain. If you stub your toe you instantly feel the pain in your toe. But there is a lot more to that than you realize. When you stub your toe a message gets sent from the toe to the brain. This message tells the brain what happened. In response the brain sends the electrical impulse back down to the toe telling it that it now hurts. That is why you feel pain. Your brain virtually creates the pain via chemicals and electrical impulses. In order to reduce the pain you might take aspirin or some other form of pain reliever. This doesn't actually go to the toe where you think the pain is coming from. Rather, the pain reliever goes to the brain and interrupts the chemical and electrical impulses that the brain is creating that makes you feel the pain. In essence, the pain you experience really is in your mind.

On a more normal day, when you aren't stubbing your toe and causing your brain to create pain, your brain will be busy creating and supervising the chemicals needed to regulate your body's functions. Everything from emotions to feeling tired, from hunger to feeling anxious, are all manifestations of the brain at work. The brain sends the feelings of hunger and the thoughts of food when the body tells it that its energy levels are low. Additionally, the brain will send feelings of drowsiness and thoughts of sleep when the body needs rest. All of these reactions are caused when certain chemicals are created and released within the brain. We don't ever pay attention to this because we have become completely used to the process. However, the importance of the brain and the impact it has on our health is all important if you want to master the art of self-healing.

As mentioned before, the number one cause of sickness is stress. This is because stress has a direct and negative impact on the brain and how it operates. When you understand that the brain regulates bodily functions then you can understand just how devastating the results of a poorly performing brain can actually be on the body. A prime example of this is the common headache. Whenever you get stressed out about a particular thing the chances are that it can give you a headache of one form or another. Sometimes this may be just a mild headache, the kind that can be eliminated simply by rubbing your temples. However, sometimes this headache can take the far more sinister form of a migraine. In each case the pain is not actually the result of physical trauma, rather it is the result of a high level of stress being put on the brain. This can begin to reveal the true nature of sickness itself. After all, if pain can be the result of something seemingly non-physical, such as anxiety or stress, so too, other sickness and diseases be caused by non-physical conditions.

This makes even more sense when you consider that as well as being the electro-chemical command center of the body the brain is also the seat of intellect and perhaps the soul. If we take the liberty of combining the intellect and soul into the entity called *mind* then this will make even more sense. After all, the mind is where all emotions and thoughts are experienced. Therefore, if the mind is in the brain then stress itself is experienced in the brain. This means that the brain reacts directly to the stress, creating electro-chemical reactions that affect the body in many different ways. While headaches are the most relatable example of this phenomenon they are certainly not the only example available. In fact, every single physical reaction to stress, including indigestion, fatigue, high blood pressure, panic attacks, adrenaline rushes, headaches and even acne can be traced to the brain. This means that stress alone can throw the chemical balance of the brain out of whack to a point where the brain creates a physiological reaction that is detrimental to your body's health. And this is just the beginning.

Since the brain is responsible for governing all bodily functions when the brain starts to act in a negative way then all bodily functions will begin to suffer. Not only will the brain create problems commonly associated with stress, but it will also begin to underperform in other vital areas. One main area directly impacted by stress is the body's immune system. Medical research has shown that stress significantly reduces the body's ability to fight sickness and disease. As a result, the higher the stress levels of a person is the more likely they are to get sick. This can manifest itself in basic ways, such as the common cold, flu or viral infections. Additionally, a person who is suffering from stress or anxiety will usually take longer to heal from cuts or abrasions to the skin, as well as broken bones, sprains or the like. In fact many medical facilities stress the importance of relaxation and de-stressing to their patients as this helps to speed up the recovery process in all cases.

The fact that stress directly affects the human body should come as no real shock. After all, many religions have treated sickness as a punishment by the divine. Sin is often associated with sickness, resulting in many traditions teaching that a person will be free from physical afflictions when they correct their behaviors. Needless to say, this can become a very dangerous mindset as it can create the idea that people are to blame for any sickness and disease that they suffer. This is not only a horrible notion to contemplate, but it can also be very counter intuitive regarding the process of self-healing. The last thing a person who is seeking power over their body needs is guilt. However, the correlation between stress and wrongdoing may in fact have a lot to do with this ancient connection between sin and sickness. Since guilt can be a significant cause of stress it makes sense that a person feeling guilty may be more susceptible to physical symptoms of stress, including sickness, due to a weakened immune system.

The question is how can knowing that stress causes sickness be useful in terms of self healing? Simply put, when it comes to sickness the old axiom 'an ounce of prevention is worth a pound of cure' is very applicable. Just as a healthy diet can prevent a great many sicknesses, so too, a healthy state of mind can do the same. By removing stress whenever and wherever possible you will ensure that your brain operates to its maximum potential. This will result in all bodily functions being healthy and strong, not least of which being the immune system. Therefore, take stock over the things that cause you anxiety and stress and actively seek to remove these things from your life. If watching the news causes you distress, which it would for any sane person in this day and age, then consider unplugging for a while. The world will be just fine if you ignore it for a time. Think of stress like calories. Just as you would cut out high calorie foods if you wanted to lose weight, so too you should cut out any input that creates stress if you want to create a healthier mindset. By reducing stress you will not only be able to prevent many sicknesses and diseases, but you will also be able to heal yourself from any current ailments simply by restoring your body to its natural balance. Again, the body is designed to restore itself, and the brain is in charge of that process. Therefore, to reduce and eliminate stress is to restore the self-healing nature of your body.

Perhaps that is one of the most important things to realize. This isn't about you creating some sort of higher reality in your life. Rather, this is about restoring yourself to your proper design. By nature, you are designed to be a self-regulating, self-healing physical being. When your physical wellbeing is suffering it means that you aren't living up to your design. All you have to do is to remove the things that are causing you harm in order to achieve a

144

complete and total state of wellbeing. By avoiding the things that cause unnecessary stress and anxiety you can return to that state of self-regulation and self-healing. It is your inherent design—the state you were intended to enjoy while on this Earth.

Conclusion

Thank you again for reading this book!

I hope this book was not only able to help you develop a healthy and happy life, but was also able to pave the way for a brighter future not just for you, but for people that surround you.

The next step is to follow these instructions and continue them even after you heal yourself. Do notice how all the points in each chapter are varied and suggestive, which means I am giving you the liberty to choose and follow your inhibition exactly as I told you in chapter 2! And remember, this may seem like a challenge but then again "if it doesn't challenge you it doesn't change you!"

Finally, if you enjoyed this book, then I'd like to ask you for a favor. Would you be kind enough to leave a review for this book on Amazon? It'd be greatly appreciated!

Please go to the below link to post your review

lrd.to/Master

Thank you and Good Luck!

Here are some of my other books.

Align your Mind, Body, and Soul - Experience Abundance of "Spiritual Energy" Through Chakra Healing & Chakra Meditation.

Get this awesome book and find balance in your life.

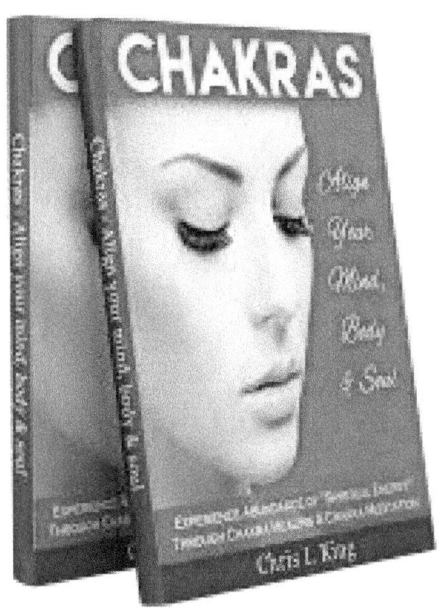

Please go to the below website to get your copy

lrd.to/Chakras

Your Ultimate Guide to Unleashing Your Psychic Abilities.

Written for anyone who wants to practice and use the power of knowing the past and the present, as well as predict the future.

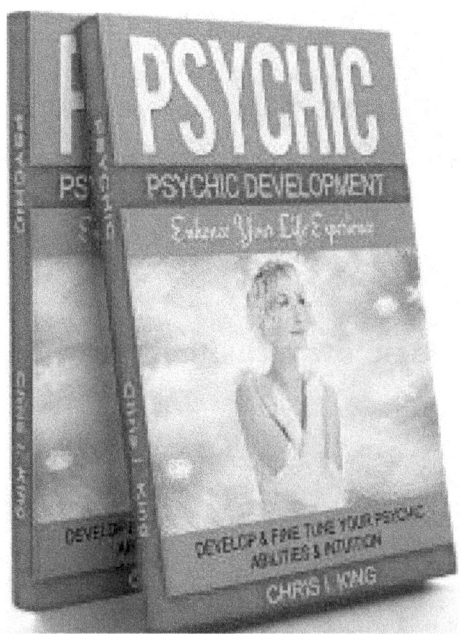

Please get your copy on the below website

lrd.to/Psychic

Happy Reading!